THE APPLICATION OF HOLISTIC LIFE COACHING TO MST
(Military Sexual Trauma)

By
Dr. Donna E. King

DEDICATION

This book is dedicated to:
My Lord and Savior Jesus Christ;
My mother, Anita C. Bowen, for her unconditional love when I was in my valley at the lowest point of my life. "Love, peace and joy!"; my sisters – Bernadine, Bernadette, Loretta, Laureen and LaVerne – for being my motivators; my pastor, John I. Caples of Jesus Name Apostolic Church, who gave me the strength and spiritual backbone to travel on this journey; and, to my other family and friends who gave me the encouragement to go on. I thank you all.

Namaste

THE APPLICATION OF HOLISTIC LIFE COACHING TO MST
(Military Sexual Trauma)

Written By
Dr. Donna E. King

Edited By
Mylia Tiye Mal Jaza

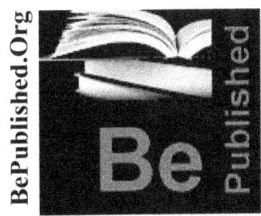

The Application of Holistic Life Coaching to MST (Military Sexual Trauma)
Copyright © 2013, Dr. Donna E. King
All Rights Reserved.

ISBN 10: 1484962869   ISBN 13: 978-1484962862

Author Contact Info
Dr. Donna E. King
donity1@sbcglobal.net
info@drdonnaeking.com
www.drdonnaeking.com

Self-Publishing Associate
BePublished.Org - Chicago, IL
mari@bepublished.org
Dr. Mary M. Jefferson
P.O. Box 8324
Jackson, MS 39284
(972) 880-8316

Imprint of Record
CreateSpace dba On-Demand Publishing
7290-B Investment Drive
Charleston, SC 29418

First Edition
Printed in the United States of America.
Recycled Paper Encouraged.

4

TABLE OF CONTENTS

Chapter	Page
1 - Introduction …………………………………..	7
2 - Review of Literature ………..………………..	11
3 - Methods …………………...……….…..……	27
4 - Findings ……………………………….…...	39
5 - Discussion ……………….…......…………..	80
6 - Summary and Conclusions …………………	89
Bibliography ………………….…..……………	95
Appendix …………………………………....	100

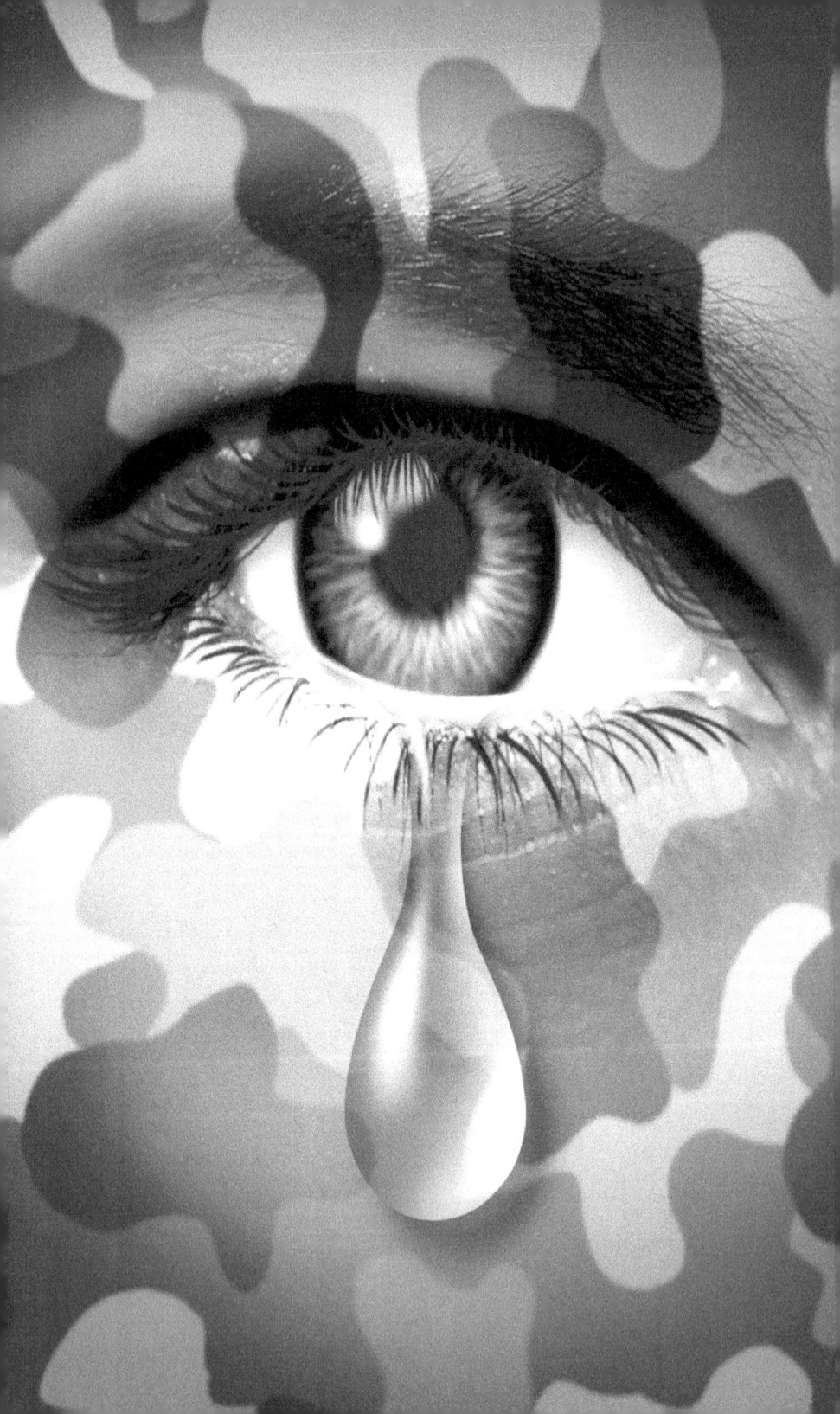

CHAPTER 1
INTRODUCTION

I grew up in New York, the eldest of six girls. My childhood years were very interesting; my mother had me, then twins and triplets, all girls. We all attended Catholic school and, by the time I reached the eighth grade, I began my search for a more spiritual feeling. Something in my being told me there was more.

My cousins attended a Pentecostal church, so I asked my mom if I could start going with them after I attended mass early Sunday morning. She said yes. I started attending church with them pretty regularly and I really enjoyed it. I learned all of the books in the Bible and could recite them so well; boy was I proud of myself.

I was blessed to have one child (a daughter) and to have a granddaughter and grandson today. I am very grateful because, had the military sexual trauma that I will describe in this dissertation taken place first, I would not have a child or any grandchildren today.

After completing high school, I entered the military; this is where I gleaned my knowledge about MST (Military Sexual Trauma). From an early age, I knew I wanted to be in the military, and I proudly served in the Army. While in the military, just going out with a few girlfriends to a club on a military installation was where my experience began. I will not elaborate on what took place, as I am still learning to cope with the demons that haunt me on a daily basis.

This contribution to Holistic Life Coaching in the area of MST will hopefully help others who are suffering in silence as I did for many, many years. However, wanting to be a Holistic Life Coach, I am working on healing myself so that I may best help others.

The Holy Bible teaches (Luke 4:23) "Physician heal thyself" – which, to me, means let me work on me before I venture out and try to help others.

I remember so many things I want to forget. I remember, once upon a time, I was a real person. Then, I was a soldier. Now, I am a ghost.

In my search for understanding and aspiring to obtain a higher level of consciousness, I have developed what I consider a unique and new found knowledge or insight in all I have read. My desire is to convey this knowledge and understanding in a comprehensive treatise that expresses my need for wanting to incorporate metaphysics into healing Military Sexual Trauma.

CHAPTER 2
REVIEW OF LITERATURE

I am going to list just a few of the definitions that are given to describe MST. First, the definition of MST used by the VA is U.S. Code 1720D of Title 38 cited as "psychological trauma, which in the judgment of a VA mental health professional, resulted from a physical assault of a sexual nature, battery of a sexual nature, or sexual harassment which occurred while the Veteran was serving on active duty or active duty for training." Sexual harassment is further defined as "repeated, unsolicited verbal or physical contact of a sexual nature which is threatening in character."

Second, MST is the term that the Department of Veterans Affairs uses to refer to sexual assault or repeated, threatening sexual harassment that occurred while the Veteran was in the military.

Third, MST is military sexual trauma. MST is the result of military personnel harassing, assaulting or raping of another military service member. Many symptoms are similar to PTSD (Post Traumatic Stress Disorder) and can range from minor to severe.

Just to further help the reader understand, I will give a few more excerpts from the Department of Veteran Affairs (2008) and what this trauma means to them and the methods they choose to use.

Sexual trauma that is associated with military service most often occurs in a setting where the victim lives and works. In most cases, this means that victims must continue to live and work closely with their perpetrators, often leading to an increased sense of feeling helpless, powerless, and at risk for additional victimization.

In addition, sexual victimization that occurs in this setting often means that victims are relying on their perpetrators (or associates of the perpetrator) to provide for basic needs including medical and psychological care. Similarly, because military sexual trauma occurs within the workplace, this form of victimization disrupts the career goals of many of its victims. Perpetrators are frequently peers or supervisors responsible for making decisions about work-related evaluations and promotions.

Also, victims are often forced to choose between continuing military careers, during which they are forced to have frequent contact with their perpetrators, and sacrificing their career goals in order to protect themselves from future victimization. As you can see there are so many variations to the definition, however they all mean the same thing to me.

From this point on, the author will help the reader take a short walk through the perils of sexual trauma. I will also attempt to help you understand why I feel that metaphysics and meditation can help contribute to society with my working as a Holistic Life Coach to help save the lives of people living with MST and PTSD.

Nancy Detweiler's Jesus approach to healing expresses my enlightenment and belief that prayer without meditation is devoid of meaning. She states, "preparation for prayer entails turning your attention inward and focusing on God dwelling within us, our I Am Presence. Prayer is a lifting upward of our thought energy, an elevating of our consciousness to the higher realms of existence."

www.Pathwaytoascension.com

My attempt to emphasize this was done by quoting Luke 18: 10-14. Detweiler uses Psalms in illustrating how the Psalmist described his preparation for prayer. "I will lift up mine eyes to the hills from whence cometh my help, my help comes from the Lord who made heaven and earth," she wrote in "If Jesus Is A Wayshower, What Did Show Us?" (*Nancy Detweiler, M.Ed., M.Div. Revised,* Part 8 of Series" Lord, Teach Us to Pray" http://www.pathwaytoascension.com/bible9.html).

In paraphrasing Detweiler, prayer is a compound process. This process involves a bipolar flow of energy that enjoins our physical self and our God Presence or our I Am Presence. This is a process done in solitude in a posture of total relaxation, using objective introspection of self to open one's heart and mind to the wisdom of God's answer.

Detweiler describes my paraphrasing thusly, prayer and its answer is that two-way flow of energy between our physical self and our I Am Presence. It is done in secret and not with a motive of impressing others. The power and glory are to be God's alone.

With that being said, this is how I begin my day. For me, it is not just during the day that I must meditate; because of the intrusive thoughts that I am plagued with, it is a twenty four (24) hour struggle. However, I have come a long way.

Holistic Life Coaching is based on my understanding that effective coaching is only possible when the multidimensional parts of an individual are included. B. Reque-Dragicevic in *Close to Home: A Soldier's Guide to Returning from War* writes that "an increasingly common trauma far less talked [than PTSD] about is military sexual trauma — which is experiencing sexual assault or harassment while you are in the military." (P, 72)

This is not just a women's problem. In fact, the VA reports that fifty-five percent of women and thirty-eight percent of men in the military have experienced military sexual harassment. While military sexual trauma is more common in women, over half of all veterans with military sexual trauma are men.

War has historically seen an increase in sexual assault and rape incidents for both military and war-zone populations. It's become more publicly recognized in war-zone civilian populations (mass gang rapes were widely reported during the Bosnian war and rape has traditionally been a way to violate an enemy population), but rarely do we hear about sexual assault among our own soldiers.

If you have experienced a sexual violation during war that has left you "just not feeling the same" since, please know that you are not alone. Most victims of military sexual trauma will never report it. Whether or not you call it rape doesn't matter. What happened to you wasn't right and it wasn't your fault; and no, you couldn't have prevented or stopped it.

I believe Dr. David Burns in his book, *"The Feeling Good Handbook,"* describes it best. He speaks of the five techniques to use as tools for better communication and thinking. The first principle of cognitive therapy is that all of our moods are created by our thoughts. We feel the way we do right now because of the thoughts we are thinking at this moment. The moment we have a certain thought and believe it, we will have an immediate emotional response.

Dr. P.L. Masters shows us the prominent role of the conscious mind. He states: "the simplest and most direct way is through positive thinking – not allowing negative thoughts to become part of one's mental subconscious reality. In metaphysics, we try to condition the subconscious so that it will think positively, while rejecting negative, self-destructive thoughts," (*Master's Degree Level Lessons*, Vol#1, Page 18). After reading this, I started to use these techniques on myself.

Mary Baker Eddy, through her belief of Christian Science, is a true proponent of the holistic approach to both physical and emotional healing that the mind governs the body not partially but wholly.

Teresa Brennan's theory of *The Transmission of Affect,* the idea that one can soak up someone else's depression or anxiety or sense the tension in a room, is familiar. "Negative energy," "dumping" suggests that the masculine subject is constructed through transferring his negative emotions to a feminized other; the victim is both burdened with his toxic affect and depleted of her vital energies. This process characterizes sexual abuse, including rape, battery, and incest. The victim feels possessed, consumed, trashed, drained, and "dirtied."

As ecological feminist theory suggests, this process is mirrored in masculine-identified abuse of the feminine-identified elemental environment. This is very true, speaking from my own experience. I felt like I was so dirty, every fiber of my being was destroyed because, to me, my life was over and I did not want to live. All of my hopes and dreams had been taken away.

Psychologist Robert Grant conveyed this message: "Traumatic experience can break a person, destroying trust in God and the world. Or it can provide a spiritual opening - a crack that opens the way to a deeper sense of life's meaning."
http://www.ptsdsupport.net/gazette.html

At first I just wanted to die. As time went on I gained a spiritual opening, it became all I had to hold on to in order to keep my sanity.

R.J. Woolger, in his book *Healing Your Past Lives: Exploring the Many Lives of the Soul* and also in his in his article *"Past Life Therapy, Trauma Release and the Body,"* mentions D. Tansley's use of Alice Bailey's version of the yogic subtle body theory. This is one I have found especially valuable, particularly since it defines, very clearly, three distinct levels of subtle energy and shows how they interpenetrate.

Bailey used the Yogic terms for these subtle bodies but in an approachable fashion. In summary and in descending order, containing each other like Russian eggs, they are:

1. The Mental Body: This very broad energy field is the most subtle of the three and is the focus of all powerful mental contents or fixed thoughts. These thoughts may be conscious or unconscious and can radically influence an individual's overall life patterns or self-image (e.g. "I'll never make it." "Don't trust people," etc.). Such thoughts can be the residues of past negative life experiences. They do not incessantly affect the lower bodies, but if they do, their influence is extremely strong.

2. The Emotional Body (sometimes called the astral body): This energy field adheres closely to the physical body by a radius of about two to four feet and is the focus of the feeling residues from past events like the mental body, including past

lives. These feelings may be sadness, rage, apathy, disappointment, etc. This energy level may be strongly affected by negative thoughts from the mental body. Physically, it is denser than the mental body. When its feeling contents become highly charged and not released, it will affect the lower etheric energy body adversely.

3. The Etheric Body: This could be called "the physical memory field" because in it resides all the painful subtle memory traces of physical trauma -- whether lesions, fractures, tumors, amputations, wounds or diseases. These are traces that Patanjali, in the Yoga Sutras, called the klesas or "sufferings" carried by the subtle body. The "phantom limb" phenomenon experienced by amputees is a well-known example of how a residual memory of trauma can be held in the etheric body.

The important principle that I gleaned from this highly condensed description is that there is a descending order of influence from higher to lower among these three bodies. In my case, the following pattern can be discerned:

1. The unconscious thought: "I am in danger" (mental level) makes me feel perpetually anxious;

I am always feeling like I have to guard myself from some impending danger. (emotional level);

2. My perpetual anxiety (emotional level) creates constant tension in my stomach region. (etheric level);

3. The constant tension in my stomach (etheric level) affects the gastrointestinal system to produce acid reflux (physical level).

Cyndi Dale's, *The Subtle Body: An Encyclopedia of Your Energetic Anatomy*, gives a greater insight into understanding how the energy levels of the body really operate. It is a comprehensive encyclopedia devoted to the critical world of our invisible anatomy, where so much of healing actually occurs.

In *Queendom*, E.M. Ellis suggests that there are "three sequences in reaction to rape: a short-term, intermediate and long-term reaction. Short-term reaction is characterized by a range of traumatic symptoms, such as somatic complaints, sleep disturbance and nightmares, fear, suspiciousness, anxiety, major depression and impairment in social functioning."

http://www.artcbt.com/RapeTraumaSyndromeTreatment.html

Cohen and Roth found that both approach and avoidance coping strategies were negatively related to recovery. However, since rape is an attack on one of the most vulnerable aspects of a person, it is very hard to cope with for nearly every woman. Therefore, the psychological strength is not the only factor, but it must not even be the most important one.

Renner suggests that the victim is caught in a "no win" situation. If the woman decides to fight back at the time of the assault, she is more likely to receive social support from her family and friends;

and police and medical personnel are more likely to believe her. On the other hand, she has to pay a price for this support. First, she is more likely to be injured from the assault. Thus, she would need medical attention, the police would be further involved, and she would have to give her explanation to many people. Her immediate crisis would be, then, very severe.

I always felt my circumstance to be a no-win situation. There was no one I could tell, without feeling like dirt. The "what if" question was always there looming in the dark. You would think, maybe I could tell this or that person. But no matter how close they were, I could not, would not, do it.

CHAPTER 3
METHODS

Since all veterans that I have worked and spoken with agreed that MST and PTSD are symptoms of a separation from the soul, I very often suggest using metaphysics and meditation to call the soul back at some point. This can be a transformational experience for the veterans, and they report a sense of peace and belonging, reconnecting with self, and releasing of the deep loneliness inside. This is a moment when metaphysics can become very spiritual, and I make sure that works with the Veteran's belief system.

However, so far, I have always seen a deep understanding beyond what I had expected with all of my fellow trauma victims about the loss of the soul, so I feel safe to suggest meditation. Even though I believed that my soul was gone, and it hurt to live like that, I chose to open up to the possibility that my soul was hiding in a safe place, waiting for me to call on it to return.

Even though I felt that my soul left me a long time ago, I allowed myself to feel safe and prepared for its return. Even though I felt so lost and lonely, I didn't know what had happened and how to live with it. I tell my soul now that I am safe, I made it through, and I can't wait for it to return to me. Now, I just meditate on:

"I am calling my soul back."

"I can't wait for it to return."

"I am so glad that this is over now."

"What a nightmare it has been. Glad it won't continue to be!"

"I remember the years when I didn't know if I was going to make it through, but I realize now that I am getting there."

"I must have it in me."

"I must be a survivor!"

"I have what it takes to survive even the toughest situations!"

"And, I deserve to be proud of myself and call my soul back – in a way that works for me!"

Meditation elevates my vibration even higher and allows for me to realize on all levels that I am safe and can be at peace with the here and now. I gave Dr. Masters' teachings and metaphysics a chance, and I was thrilled with the results. Within four sessions, I felt some release of all the associated trauma, emotions, and obsessions that interfered with my sleep. Sleep became a little more easy and gentle activity, at times free from worry and fretting.

Today, I let my body tell me when to sleep instead of rigorously following a clock. Sleep today is more of a joy at times, so I am still working to fully release myself and feel safe. I will have some more clean-ups to do in relation to my military experiences and the chronic physical pain that I feel. But this is a great start.

It's my deep-seated belief that women veterans who suffer military sexual trauma risk being twice betrayed: once by their perpetrator in uniform and once by the system itself, which should be doing a much better job of protecting them from a problem that's too apparent, widespread, and part of the actual culture to pretend that it doesn't exist.

From the various readings on the true essence of Metaphysics, a new door opened to how totally encompassing metaphysics is and I finally really realized what the term Holistic means; the discipline of metaphysics encompasses all aspects of reality. Using the simple example of drug addiction, the truth is that a client has a need for a drug. That is a truth, but the reality is that although the addiction and the addictive behavior exist, he/she can change that behavior by eliminating the addiction by curing the source of the addiction (not the symptoms of the addiction, but the underlying causes of the illness of the addiction).

Speaking from experience, it is a process which takes many years to learn to change your thought patterns and ways of doing things. In my experience, many Veterans and people with PTSD symptoms never feel that they arrive in the present. They keep reliving their trauma from years ago, and their minds function as if the trauma was still happening. So, they feel threatened in their daily life and surround themselves with weapons and defense mechanisms.

As I begin to see the changes in me, the different levels of consciousness that I obtain and the changes in my state of mind and being, I slowly realize that it is a good change and it can possibly help others. Using Dr. David Burns' *Five Techniques for Communication* allowed me to communicate better when incorporated with Dr. Masters' teachings. I will list them and show how they helped me and others with whom I shared the knowledge.

The five techniques are triple column, disarming, empathy, active listening, and descripting. The first principle of cognitive therapy is that all of our moods are created by our thoughts. We feel the way we do right now because of the thoughts we are thinking at this moment. The moment we have a certain thought and believe it, we will have an immediate emotional response.

In mine and the case of others I interviewed, having constant intrusive thoughts kept us in a state of panic. Using metaphysics, meditation and affirmations, we were able to take ourselves to another level of feeling some relief.

The Triple Column Technique is useful for talking back to your internal critic (the little voice inside our heads that criticizes our behavior). Automatic Thoughts (negative thoughts) are the negative ways that we think of ourselves and others. They are self-criticisms. Cognitive Distortion/Feelings (bent reality) are the ways our automatic thoughts are twisted, bent out of shape, or blown out of proportion. Rational Responses (examples/evidence) are positive thoughts and are the means by which you shoot down automatic thoughts.

Using the Triple Column Technique to talk back to our inner critic is where the affirmations were very useful. When we were criticizing ourselves, we could now talk back in a positive way, i.e., "I am a lovable person who is loved by others; I am appreciated by others, I am safe; and so it is, I can make change because I am one with the Divine Spirit, I am one with God, I am a divine creation of the Universal Spirit. These are just a few examples of the affirmations we use and are told to boldly speak back. These were our rational/positive responses.

Disarming: This is the most difficult and the most powerful listening skill. You find some truth in what the other person is saying and agree with them, even if you think that what they are saying is wrong. During the disarming sessions, we laughed and we cried. As stated by Dr. Burns, it was one of the most difficult times we went through, however we learned and we are still learning to overcome.

Empathy: You put yourself in the other person's shoes and try to see the world through his or her eyes. This was a very easy task for those of us that suffered trauma, but for many of those who have not, they could not even begin to imagine what we went through.

Active Listening: This is displayed by letting the person know that you are really paying attention to what they are saying. Repeating what they have said will let them know that you have heard them. Although we struggled with active listening at first, we overcame the obstacles with constant practice, e.g., "I understand you said that you were very afraid to go out." With your repeating, the other person begins to feel better because they know they are really being heard. So we began to repeat and use an affirmation such as, "I understand you said that you were very afraid to go out. We all feel that way and we will overcome."

DESC Scripting is unique approach for dealing with interpersonal conflict by helping you to be more assertive. It will help you to analyze conflicts, determine your needs and rights, and propose a resolution to the conflict. Through metaphysics, meditation, and spirituality, we will resolve our conflicts.

In teaching or counseling, my technique will first ask the questions Detweiler asked of herself: "Does the client believe in the Bible, does the client believe that the teachings bring inner peace, compassion, joy, and overall permanent

enhancement to his/her life?" (Part 8 of Series
"Lord, Teach Us to Pray"

http://www.pathwaytoascension.com/bible9.html,)

Does the religious philosophy that the client
adheres to offer him/her the opportunity to serve
him/herself and others? If the answer is yes, then
our search for discovery will be much easier. If
not, my purpose is to lead the clients to the true
discovery of truth for themselves.

The writings of Detweiler and my other
readings have encouraged my belief that
metaphysics as well as the Bible is indeed a true
manual and guide to confronting life's problems.
The concept of an unbiased quest for true positive
self-actualization can only be realized through a
holistic approach to physical as well as emotional
health.

Understanding that repair of the physical and emotional damage that afflicts man in general can be achieved through growth and recognition of each of our own particular I Am Self (or God-Head), I submitted my metaphysics system of treating disease trauma to a practical test. Could it really rid me of my suffering? Since then, this system has gradually gained ground and has proven itself, whenever I used the knowledge I obtained from Dr. Masters and others, to be a most effective curative practice for myself and other veterans that trusted me to help them.

CHAPTER 4
FINDINGS

The understanding of how to use all I have gleaned from my present course of study has led me to believe that metaphysics is the true key to solving life's problems. "The one who believes in me will also do the works that I do and in fact will do greater works than these, because I am going to the Father," John 14:12 reads.

To actually see this concept in practice, one only has to look at the so-called drug problem that is currently plaguing societies all over the world. Heretofore, doctors or counselors attempted to cure the addictions simply by alleviating the physical body of the need or cravings for the drug. This treatment failed miserably because no one thought to treat the problems that caused the addiction in the first place. The lack of a truly holistic approach to the cure causes an eventual and inevitable relapse. Immediately apparent is how beneficial a holistic metaphysical approach to the illness of addiction can be. Metaphysics teaches the ill addict the true meaning of mind over matter.

Providing the knowledge of self-actualization and ridding one's self of the err of negative thinking goes a long way toward realizing the I Am Presence or the divine God-Head in each individual. Once the addict is cleansed of the drug, an emotional scrubbing of his/her essence of being and the realization and truth of what is the root of the addiction, through intelligent rationalization, is key to curing the addiction by eliminating negative behaviors.

The tools, our manual, of living metaphysics by definition - simply put - is the concept that "I think therefore I am." This allowed me to clear my mind of my addiction, since the hospital had cleared my body of the craving for drugs.

Realizing that metaphysics is the philosophy of self-realization is the key to higher self-esteem and emotional well-being.

It is easy to see to see why metaphysics is sometimes referred to as the science beyond nature. I feel as though rape is always an issue of power, not sex. Rape, sometimes also called sexual assault, can happen to both men and women of any age.

The U.S. Federal Bureau of Investigation (FBI) defines rape as: "The penetration, no matter how slight, of the vagina or anus with any body part or object, or oral penetration by a sex organ of another person, without the consent of the victim."

Rape is forced and unwanted. It's about power, not sex. A rapist uses actual force or violence — or the threat of it — to take control over another human being. Some rapists use drugs to take away a person's ability to fight back. Rape is a crime whether the person committing it is a stranger, a date, an acquaintance, or a family member. No matter how it happened, rape is frightening and traumatizing. People who have been raped need care, comfort, and a way to heal.

What Should I Do?

What's the right thing to do if you've been raped? Take care of yourself in the best way for you. For some people, that means reporting the crime immediately and fighting to see the rapist brought to justice. For others, it means seeking medical or emotional care without reporting the rape as a crime. Every person is different.

There are three things that everyone who has been raped should do:

1) Know that the rape wasn't your fault, seek medical care, and deal with your feelings. Unfortunately, rape happens too often as people deal with overwhelming feelings of god-like power, lowered inhibitions, excessive anger, lack of usual sexual release and the devaluation of human life — sexual force is often used with little outward consequence to the perpetrator. But the consequences to the victim are life-changing. If this has happened to you, you may develop PTSD from this alone, but don't be too embarrassed or humiliated to tell anyone, why? This may be the hardest part of your experience to deal with and

one that strangles you in secrecy, shame, and embarrassment.

After all, with fellow survivors coming back with missing limbs and mental shock, how can having been sexually violated compare to that? No one would believe you, would they? What would love ones think? Soldiers are supposed to be tough; how could you ever admit that you weren't strong enough to keep someone from forcing sex on you? Yet, for me, what happened has become my war, a war that no one will ever know anything about.

2) Take a deep breath, I know this is a lot for anyone who has not been through this to comprehend, forget the fact that it was not a war environment for me for a moment and realize that no matter where it happens, when, or to whom, being sexually violated always leaves a person feeling powerless, doubtful of themselves,

uncertain, unable to believe it really happened, and feeling very, very small inside. Why? Because sexual assault is about taking away your power. Sex is our most intimate and most powerful interaction with another human being. And when someone overpowers us physically and enters our bodies without our consent, we are deeply ashamed and shocked at how powerless we were.

Reque-Dragicevic (*Sexual Violence Injures the Soul,* 2008) adds that the shame, humiliation, loss of control, and shaken self-esteem affect both men and women even though each gender experiences them differently because of what we are conditioned to believe about our masculine or feminine roles in life.

Sexual violation impacts our self-image, sexuality, and our future, safe sexual experiences. The overwhelming sense of vulnerability and shame can lead to suicidal thoughts and actions. For war survivors who have been violated by one of their own, the confusion and uncertainty, not to mention potential repercussions to your military career or even survival, lead most victims to never tell anyone. Keeping your mouth shut may be the only way to survive and get back home. But once you are home, please realize that if this has happened to you, you have been affected and it's not just going to go away. It takes feeling safe to get yourself to the point where you can admit to someone that it happened. And for a lot of people, finding someone safe seems almost impossible.

The VA also reports that it has counselors at every hospital trained to assist veterans with this issue. Remember, what happened to you was a crime, not just a misfortune of war. The person who assaulted you did not have the right to do this to you under any circumstances.

3) One of the hardest parts about having been sexually traumatized can be sharing that information with a spouse or partner. It's normal to worry about how they will accept you once they know what has happened and to wonder how it will impact your intimate life together. Even though this trauma may loom large before your eyes, your partner loves you and offers more acceptance than you imagine. You are still attractive, beautiful, desirable, virile, and your partner still longs to experience sexual intimacy with you. You may struggle with feeling that you are not worth loving which is one of the ways sexual violation diminishes your own sense of power. But feelings are not facts. You are a human being worth being

loved, enjoyed, and you deserve to experience sexual intimacy in a safe and caring relationship.

Partners of sexual assault survivors may feel a sense of rage, powerlessness, guilt for not having been able to protect your loved one, and a natural reaction to want to get even with the person who has hurt the person you love. Counseling individually and as a couple can be a safe place to express what you are feeling. You can also call the Sexual Assault Hotline—it's not just for survivors; they can assist family and friends.

Remember, as long as you don't tell your partner what happened, he or she will have no way of knowing what you are feeling, worried about, remembering, or associating with your current sex life. You may have no desire to have sex because of the trauma, but how will your partner know that? If you don't share, he or she may assume that they are no longer desirable and that you've lost interest. They may easily blame themselves or you. Don't lose your relationship because you are too ashamed to share what happened. Seek a counselor who can help you decide how to share this information. Don't shut out what may be the only true source of love and support in your life. Loving partners can be incredibly patient when it comes to sex and trauma, but you have to give them the chance to understand what you are going through.

If you have been sexually traumatized, it may seem that that experience now defines who you are. Shame, guilt, self-blame, denial, rage, depression, lack of self-worth, fear of being intimate again, aversion to being touched or approached without warning, doubts about whether or not you are still desirable, or if having been raped effects your sexual orientation (it doesn't) are all normal reactions. Just remember the trauma is real and intimate, but you are not defined by what has happened to you. You are a whole person who has experienced vulnerability and powerlessness; but that experience did not change who you really are: still strong, still powerful, still in control and still able to move toward healing. Deciding to move toward healing may be the only justice you ever get for what happened. You owe it to yourself, your partner, and your children to make sure that this trauma does not take you away from them any more than it already has.

To understand what a person that has suffered MST; you actually have to walk in their shoes.

What people also fail to realize is that being in the military is not necessarily being in a war zone. A lot of times when people speak of MST they relate it to combat, not understanding that being in the military is also like working a regular civilian job, the only difference is you are in uniform.

Detweiler *Your Inner Spiritual Journey* "Your inner Spiritual Journey begins as you take responsibility for your life, meaning that you no longer walk unconsciously through life, placing the blame for events in your life onto something outside of yourself. Instead you make the conscious choice to grow holistically."

Masters, according to the basic tenets of Metaphysics you must purge yourself of all negativity including your physical body, emotions, thoughts, and intuitive awareness, such purging allows you to reach your indwelling God or the I am Presence. You in a holistic sense are the Temple in which God dwells.

Eddy, Eddy realizes that need to understand the differences between truth and reality. She notes that true emotional as well as physical healing cannot be achieved without said acknowledgement, "suffering is no less a mental condition than is enjoyment. You cause bodily sufferings and increase them by admitting their reality and continuance, as directly as you enhance your joys by believing them to be real and continuous.

When an accident happens you think or exclaim "I am hurt" your thoughts are more powerful than your words, more powerful than the accident itself, to make the injury real, Thoughts, proceeding from the brain or from matter, are offshoots of mortal mind; they are mortal material beliefs. Ideas are spiritual, harmonious, and eternal. Beliefs proceed from the so-called material senses, which at one time are supposed to be substance-matter and at another are called spirits." *Science & Health*, Page 88:9-16

Metaphysics helps when meditation is used to objectively understand that truth never governs reality but in order to understand the depth of truth one must first come to grips with what is truly reality. Truth is simply the reality that a condition exists reality says true you have an addition but it is your choice to continue to be an addict.

As I begin to see the changes in me and the different levels of consciousness that I obtain and the changes in my state of mind and being, I slowly realize that it is a good change and it can possibly help others.

Dr. Anneli Driessen PhD. *Connecting with Your Multidimensional Self and Your Longing for Happiness, Ultimate Success*, gives her statements which are noted by the bullet points, I will give my opinion under her statements.

"All distress, pain and/or illness are governed by the Law of Cause and Effect."

In my opinion, this is very true. The pain I suffer daily was caused by my brutal trauma, and the effect is and was my loss of everything.

"The value of analysis and the search for 'WHY?' are often overrated. It is better to identify what is most important and to establish and follow a plan of action."

Today, I am working on identifying my situation and that of others in my position to establish a plan to holistically heal and nourish our minds and bodies so that our beings are restored.

"We need to control our minds (intellect) and not allow our minds to control us."

Through meditation, we will begin to allow our every thought to take us to a place that we deem as safe. Because of the knowledge that I have gained by experiencing trauma, I feel that I am equipping myself to deal with the problem that so many are plagued by.

> *"The issue of fear or terror cannot be resolved without addressing our relationship with God."*

This is a very true statement, for if it had not been for my strengthening my relationship with God, and meditation, I would not have progressed as much as I have.

> *"Acceptance is more important than understanding."*

It was very hard for me to accept what happened to me, however I had to allow myself to accept that yes this happened, if I didn't I would not been able to start the healing process. I did not need to understand, trying to understand was like walking through the desert without a destination. I had to let go of that search in order to gain acceptance.

"The individual's process of spiritual development and maturity has two focuses, the inner journey and serving others."

Yes my focus is to heal myself, and, during this process, focus on what I need to do to serve others in the field of Holistic Life Coaching.

I took each one of these points into account, and applied them to me, I asked myself each question, and metaphysically answered them one by one. I was amazed as I began to answer the questions and use them as a part of my healing, seeking to bring unity to body, mind and soul.

G.F. Rhoades held that the definition of the disassociation comes from trauma, how trauma and dissociation are related. Professionals working in the area of abuse and trauma are quite familiar with dissociative processes. Clients/ Patients commonly share in the context of treatment the phenomenon of separating their thoughts and emotions from the trauma that they were experiencing and/or had experienced in the past.

This separation (dissociation) of one's thoughts, emotions and even body sensations are commonly seen in traumatic disorders such as Post Traumatic Stress Disorder (PTSD). In addition, patients who arc diagnosed with a dissociative disorder are often discovered to have trauma in their background. The apparent co-existence of trauma and dissociation has led many therapists to note that "you can't have trauma without dissociation and that you can't have dissociation without trauma." There are always exceptions to this noted co-existence of trauma and dissociation, but nevertheless the phenomenon is quite commonly reported to therapists. There has even been discussion within the diagnostic community of possibly having Post Traumatic Stress Disorder (PTSD) listed as a dissociative disorder and thus removed from the DSM-IV category of Anxiety Disorders.

The definition Rhoades gives speaks to the trauma that I and others I have interviewed live on a daily basis. Disassociation definitely comes with trauma. You come to a place where you are always making an unconscious attempt at self-protection against an overwhelming and traumatic experience as a result from severe and prolonged maltreatment or sexual abuse.

Dissociation, wherein painful reality is transformed into a bad dream, is one of the most effective means to deal with all rapes and tortures, sadness, loneliness, grief, depression, suicides and the like. Just as a traumatized victim of an horrific and terrifying event makes the experience unreal in order to cope with the ordeal, the sages and seers – gurus and god-men/ goddess-women, the masters and messiahs, the saviors and saints – have desperately done precisely this thing (during what is sometimes called "the dark night of the soul"). Mystics have been transmogrifying the real world "reality" into an unreal "Greater Reality" via the epiphenomenal imaginative/intuitive facility born of the psyche, which is formed by the instinctual passions genetically endowed by blind nature for survival purposes.

Such disassociation is a psychotic sickness culturally institutionalized into a head-in-the-sand escapist "solution" to all the ills of humankind, hence the divine perpetuation of all the misery and mayhem across the millennia through a belief in maya / samsara / karma or some-such metaphysical fantasy being the cause of such aberrant behavior. Mysticism is nothing more and nothing less than a frantic coping-mechanism, institutionalized into a cultural metaphysics over thousands and thousands of years, especially if accompanied by dissociative states such as "derealisation" or "alternate personality disorder" and others.

It is also known as "disassociation," or "dissociative identity disorder." Dissociative reactions are attempts to escape from excessive trauma, tension and anxiety by separating off parts of personality function from the rest of cognition as an attempt to isolate something that arouses anxiety and gain distance from it.

I feel that, in normal everyday life, mild and temporary dissociation is sometimes difficult to distinguish from repression and isolation, and is a relatively common and normative device used to escape from severe emotional tension and anxiety. Temporary episodes of transient estrangement and derealisation are often experienced by normal persons when they first feel the initial impact of bad news, for instance. Everything suddenly looks strange and different, things seem unnatural and distant, events can be indistinct and vaporous, and often the person feels that they themselves are unreal and everything takes on a dream-like quality. Normal dissociation becomes abnormal when the once mild or transient expedient becomes too intense, lasts too long, or escapes from a person's control and leads to a separation from the surroundings, which seriously disturbs object relations. In object estrangement, the once familiar world of ordinary objects – the world of people, things and events – seems to have undergone a disturbing and often indescribable change.

Peter Levine, PhD, quotes Freud. "We are miserable because of our traumatic histories and that we can cure our neurosis through talk (reliving and understanding). With this cure, the most we can hope for is ordinary unhappiness (therapeutic goal)."
http://www.extatica.com/articles/Levine_P_HealingSacred Wound_1.htm.

I found this to be very true as it pertained to me. There is also a metaphysical viewpoint: When we are born, we come in not as blank slates but as "spirits" with a "blue print" for life. To unfold this "code," to materialize this "seed" as a physical "flesh" reality, we are given certain challenges and ordeals. In many metaphysical systems, it is said that we pick the situations in our lives and even our parents to actuate this unfolding. In other words, we unconsciously chose our parents and our life events in order to work through our "karma" and learn the lessons that will open our eyes to our soul's purpose. This process of embodiment is what gives our life direction and meaning. It may be a surprise to you but there are many more people on the planet that believe this view than the psychological one.

The skill we need to cultivate to transform traumatic experience is the capacity to feel our bodily sensations as they are. That means feeling sensations through to completion, in the now, without undue judgment or interpretation. This means truly feeling the feelings as they are, not suppressing them or exaggerating them. Usually we fuel sensations, inflaming them into emotions without really having any idea that this is what we are doing. What we want to avoid is our lifelong identification becoming an altar to our wounds, as precious to us as they may be. Instead, our wounds can be merely a starting point for healing, a way to begin to reclaim the temple of our bodies. The handling of the topic of sexual trauma and abuse in our society is deeply disturbing. We are now seeing scientific research showing the detrimental effect of abuse and trauma.

As Peter Levine points out, not only do psychological symptoms develop, there is now clear evidence that there can be interference with brain development and the suppression of the immune system. I would say that the only thing more appalling than the state of mental health and unnecessary suffering in our country is its treatment – or rather lack of it. Trauma and sexual abuse is one of our most important human and societal problems. It needs to be studied by free, unbiased scientific investigation rather than polarized by hysteria and politics. People are tragically hurt by sexual trauma and we need the scientific study and the compassionate application of metaphysics, spirituality, and meditation to add to the knowledge and the understanding, prevention, and healing of trauma.

The testimony of many survivors of sexual abuse reveals that healing from toxic dumping and the ensuing disconnection induced by sexual violence can be enabled in two linked ways. First of all, survivors can refuse to take on the unwanted affect. Moreover, they can energetically affirm and reconnect with elemental forces in the self and in the world.

R. Grant, on his website http://www.ptsdsupport.net/gazette.html, had the following thing to say: "Trauma has a way of finding us, and it has a power that is like nothing else." All this pain is like a refiner's fire that purifies us, if the process can be monitored and people are given enough support. Grant talked about the "dark grace" of traumatic experience, relating it to historical figures. St. Francis of Assisi was a man of privilege whose war experience turned him toward a life of poverty and service. Nelson Mandela's imprisonment became a forge for spiritual strength and political commitment. "And Christ suffered right up to the very end," said

Grant, who is convinced that great human resiliency can arise out of the most terrible circumstances.

Sexual Abuse Survivor - Is There Hope?

If you are a sexual abuse survivor, you have survived a terrible ordeal and are perhaps looking for some understanding and some peace of mind. I do not have all the answers, but I am a sexual abuse survivor and I can identify with the feelings you are experiencing. I have finally found peace of mind, and I would like to share with you some thoughts on how to overcome this unimaginable pain.

Do you know why you're a survivor? Some may call it fate, survival of the fittest, mental or emotional fortitude, or divine intervention. What is it for you?

Sexual Abuse Survivor - Accepting The Past

Sexual abuse survival involves facing the past abuse, accepting the fact that it happened. No matter what type of sexual abuse (whether incest or by a stranger) or how tragic its consequences, acceptance of the past is vital. Accepting the past is an essential step toward not only surviving, but to overcoming. Examine your past, with a trained professional if possible. Look at how you coped with the abuse while it was occurring.

What were your thoughts?
Did you feel anger, hatred, or melancholy?
Did you blame yourself or perhaps feel guilty (or unclean)?
Did you turn inward, living in your own world?
Did you tell someone?

Did that person ignore you?

Did you ignore the abuse and hope it would go away?

Did you pray to God and ask Him to intercede, but the abuse continued?

How did you feel about yourself? About others?

Were there trust issues? If so, with whom?

Were there problems with authority?

Were you distant and aloof, perhaps shy - struggling to communicate like other children?

Or, did you hide by being outgoing when you were really in a state of denial?

Maybe you were afraid to turn inward and deal with the onslaught of feelings and thoughts. Maybe you just didn't know what to do or how you felt. Not surprisingly, what happened to us in the past is often carried into the present.

Sexual Abuse Survivor - Living In The Present

If you're a sexual abuse survivor, how are things going now? As a survivor of military sexual trauma, I confess that I struggle with the effects of sexual abuse – feelings of anger, hatred, sadness, guilt, and shame toward my abuser and indirectly toward myself. Sometimes these feelings and thoughts can get in the way, interfering with other relationships. As a sexual abuse survivor, do you experience similar feelings? Do you ever wonder why me, what did I ever do to deserve the abuse? If so, you are not alone.

Unfortunately, these feelings and thoughts do not magically disappear. From personal experience and from talking with other adult survivors of sexual abuse, I've discovered we share and exhibit similar thoughts and feelings yet struggle to find an outlet. As a survivor, I simply want to be heard and understood. I want someone I can identify with. I want to be told that I am okay.

When a person has been abused sexually, thoughts like *I'm not ok* and *I will never be okay* seem to become ingrained in the psyche. In addition, there are often problems with self-acceptance, guilt, condemnation, feelings of never measuring up, and so on. Those feelings are incorrect. We are okay, and we can live a life of victory!

A proactive approach to dealing with past abuse involves getting help and taking an introspective look at what happened. Tragically, many sexual abuse survivors choose to avoid help. The confusion of unresolved sexual abuse can lead some people to go from victim to perpetrator. Or the survivor learns to cope through self-abuse, like drugs and alcohol, or develops an addiction to sex or pornography. Many abuse survivors believe they cannot get past what happened to them.

If the abuse came from the same sex, this may unfortunately lead to later interaction with same sex. If the abuse was perpetrated by someone of the opposite sex, such as a father and daughter, the daughter often seeks to fill this void through promiscuity. She is really looking for love, and has learned that she will find it through sexual activity. Of course, she does not find love, but heartache and sometimes more abuse or even disease. These lies can only lead to shattered hearts and lives.

If the need or void is not dealt with proactively, the abuse often survives in the survivor. Shadows of the abuse live on in various forms, because the abuse victim looks for satisfaction in the wrong ways or places. Having never known genuine love, the abuse survivor can only imitate love in return. Is there a way to overcome the past? I believe there is.

Sexual Abuse Survivor - Can Life Be Worth Living?

As a sexual abuse survivor, you may be asking, "Can I really move past just surviving and have a life worth living?" The answer is, "Yes! Yes you can!"

You may have heard the phrase: "If it feels good, do it." Perhaps that is how you have been living your life. You are at a standstill, just doing what makes you feel good, loved and accepted. Maybe that still involves the abuse or some attribute of the abuse. This does not have to be your life!

Maybe you're already beginning to realize that there is more to life than what happened yesterday. As a sexual abuse survivor, I've known emptiness. I know what it feels like to have a deep need for love and acceptance.

Blaise Pascal, a philosopher from the age of enlightenment, determined that there is a God-shaped hole, or vacuum, inside every human being that can only be filled by God. You may have heard stories of sex abuse survivors whose lives have been changed. Maybe you even know someone like that, and you long to be like them. You want to move beyond just coping with the past – you want to be changed! You long for a life of victory.

Sexual Abuse Survivor - Understanding The Longings In Your Soul

That longing you feel is the hole or the void that Pascal mentioned. Only God can fill that vacuum with His unconditional love and acceptance. What's more, He longs to do just that! God became a man in Jesus Christ and lived among humans, so He can identify with us in our humanity.

He calls us His beloved and wants us to experience His love. In the Bible, we read 1 John 3:1, which says, "How great is the love the Father has lavished on us, that we should be called children of God! And that is what we are! The reason the world does not know us is that it did not know him." God accepts us just as we are when we come to Him.

Sexual Abuse Survivor - How To Move from Surviving to Overcoming

As a sexual abuse survivor, you can overcome! Isn't that exciting news? How does overcoming work? For starters, God promises us that when we come to Him, we get a brand new beginning. In Jesus Christ, we become new creations! Second Corinthians 5:17 says, "Therefore, if anyone is in Christ, he is a new creation; the old has gone, the new has come!"

The Word of God says in Jesus Christ we are overcomers: "Do not be overcome by evil, but overcome evil with good" (Romans 12:21). God has already done the work for us, and He loves us just as we are. As a sexual abuse survivor, you have been through a lot. Learning to live as a new creation is like a toddler learning to walk. The toddler takes it one step at a time.

Physically, we remain injured and will carry the scars as long as we live. But God promises He is there and will never leave us. "Never will I leave you; never will I forsake you" (Hebrews 13:5). He is there when our minds recall situations, and when our minds, wills, and emotions are in darkness and despair. When we suffer mental anguish and condemnation, God is there.

As sexual abuse survivors, we'll find it difficult to reconcile thoughts and feelings regarding love and acceptance. Because of our past, we'll know feelings that combat, tear, and rip the heart and soul apart. No one should have to experience what we have been through. But there is hope.

Because God sent His Son to die for us (John 3:16), we can know that we have value and worth. As a sexual abuse survivor, this concept is hard to wrap the mind around – but it's necessary if we're going to move from a survivor to an overcomer. The essence of overcoming is realizing that love and acceptance are essential to our healing. We can't do this on our own. In fact, it's impossible! Matthew 19:26 says, "With man this is impossible, but with God all things are possible."(AllAboutLifeChallenges.org, 2002 - 2012)

Because there seems to be an awakening and embracing of Metaphysics in our society, emotional walls and religious barriers are coming down as people who formerly held fast to one doctrine or dogma are beginning to accept and affirm ancient belief systems. This faith is causing a change in lifestyle for many people. Those who never considered themselves a religious churchgoer are now finding comfort and healing through energy work, spiritual readings, holistic seminars, and new age products. This is effecting how humans treat themselves, one another, animals, and the environment.

There are seven major chakras or energy centers in the human body where energy is intercepted and transferred to every cell of the body, including the mind and spirit. The chakras can become damaged, blocked, misaligned, imbalanced, or dirty through ignorance, unhealthy lifestyles, or chemical and substance abuse. When we awaken to metaphysical knowledge and begin to access our internal energy, we can begin to heal our physical and emotional diseases.

CHAPTER 5
DISCUSSION

It is my greatest wish that my findings would affect society by healing veterans and others suffering from military sexual trauma and any other trauma. I decided to better support myself, my friends and family with the principles that changed my life to pursue a doctoral degree in Holistic Life Coaching.

As a Holistic Life Coach, my treatment would be typically 10 sessions long and the client would work with the coach to examine the impact of the trauma -- especially related to the each person's beliefs about safety, trust, power/control, esteem and intimacy. Through metaphysics, spirituality, and meditation practice assignments, the client is able to form a more realistic and balanced view of self, others, and the world, and to realize that they do not have to be controlled by the trauma any longer. By taking what I have learned in my metaphysical studies and applying it in attempts to teach or counsel, my first task is to provide an understanding of the I Am Presence, and to open an avenue to an understanding that nature or what is natural is a subjective concept. It is an ideal that should not inhibit or restrict the I Am Presence in each of us. This is not to say self-analysis, but self-realization through intellectual truth. This, of course, is a truth based on the bounds and limitations of societal reality.

Reality is not a personal concept opposed to truth; truth is a subjective concept of how one views empirical facts. Reality is the state of being limited by the boundaries of what can be changed and what cannot. At first a lot of the veterans felt that they could only be healed at the hospital, going through the old hospital ritual.

In my experimental counseling and teaching, my goal was to separate the two concepts but make the client understand how interrelated they were, as I was working with veterans and other clients to show and teach them how metaphysics is helping me to heal. So it was also understood, in my opinion, that one cannot exist without the other. I would venture to say that if given a chance, metaphysics would make a huge impact on saving the lives of those suffering from MST and PTSD.

One's metaphysics determines one's outlook/view of reality, the totality of one's ideas, one's experiences, and so on when considered as a whole. Part of this totality is one's beliefs, values, and standards.

I felt that, if Alcoholics Anonymous used some components of metaphysics in their treatment and recovery, there would be even greater success. I believed that, properly applied, those same techniques could be used in treating emotional (sexual trauma) as well as physical problems; and it worked.

MST causes emotional and physical problems; applying meditation and affirmations to myself I felt a great deal of relief.

This to me is a vital component in achieving emotional as well as physical well-being and health. When you discover truth and reality for oneself it gives you a new sense of being, you see life's situations in a different light. It is as though everything is new, you now take a different approach to events that shape, govern and present new problems in your life.

That concept is what I want to impart to clients as well as students. Metaphysics as an all-encompassing discipline which reinforced the afore mentioned ideals.

I personally feel that the need to incorporate the Metaphysical interpretation of MST is vitally important to support existing disciplines in counseling as well as teaching without such an incorporation a valuable tool is being lost, or at best misused. Clients as well as students must understand this discipline supplies a source of enlightenment that can be interpreted as beneficial, in their quest for understanding as well as self-actualization.

One's metaphysics determines one's outlook/view of reality, the totality of one's ideas, one's experiences, and so on, considered as a whole. Part of this totality is one's beliefs, values, standards, and so on. So, axiology is derivative from metaphysics. I start with metaphysics because that was how the question was formulated. It started first with the term "metaphysics" rather than "axiology." So, the "logic" of the question determines the "logic" of the answer!

This completely changes the way I view things now. By understanding more of myself, I understand more about other things. Metaphysics will define the universal laws which govern everything so that we can take greater responsibility for their correct use. By working within the laws, we progress much faster.

I find that, by combining spirituality with metaphysics, it becomes a great holistic healing tool. I find that treatment of trauma victims is still in an embryonic stage. No single therapeutic technique seems to work, so treatment is still very much a puzzle. The pieces fit together differently for every survivor. I believe that deep inside every being is an innate wise core Self that can help one reach full potential. But often we are too distracted by our external environment to hear the voice of the Self or the Soul. Trauma, abuse and violence in situations where trust and safety have been violated affect one's ability to have and sustain relationships that are satisfying and nurturing.

I feel that meditation is a spiritual practice used in many cultures for thousands of years. The techniques may vary but the intention is the same, connection and communion with the Creator or the creative source of life referred to by many as God. Meditation encourages development of higher consciousness, a part of which is greater awareness, intuition, compassion, empathy and acceptance. The practice of meditation encourages the integration of spiritual beliefs into daily life. Meditation has also been found useful in reducing stress, strengthening the immune system, and promoting good health. Meditation can increase creativity and intuition, and when used simultaneously with Holistic Life Coaching or other methods of seeking growth, it encourages mental, emotional and behavioral growth and changes.

Meditation has been helpful for me in uncovering traumatic memories, controlling habitual thoughts, anger, depression, chemical dependency and chronic pain. I would like to use metaphysics to provide an opportunity for people who have experienced emotional trauma, MST and PTSD to come together in a safe, nurturing and supportive environment. I want to encourage those who feel they would benefit from sharing their experiences of having MST and PTSD, with a focus on healing and positive support. Hopefully, this will make them feel like they are coming back to a sense of being connected with life and its opportunities for joy.

A point must be made that rape has a social nature. The victim must deal not only with rape and the impact on him/her, but also with reactions of others to it. However, if the victim does not risk injury, she/he is less likely to receive support or to be believed by police and court. She/he would be blamed by self and others for failing to resist, and would feel more guilt and have more difficulties resolving the problem in the long run.

CHAPTER 6
SUMMARY AND CONCLUSIONS

I feel that metaphysics has been and is becoming a great asset in the field of healing. How should healing and metaphysics be explored by others in the future? In my case, I experienced severe depression after my life in the military and manifested suicidal thoughts during times of crisis. I sought help from traditional counselors and medical doctors, who prescribed antidepressant medication.

However, the medication only masked the problem by covering its symptoms. Even with medication, a low level of anxiety and brain fog (confusion and inability to remain focused) continued. Additionally, while on the antidepressants, my weight had increased by 20 percent. The weight gain lowered my self-esteem, but each time I attempted to discontinue or reduce my medication, the suicidal thoughts would return and my mood disorder would worsen.

After learning about metaphysical methods of treatment, I visited an energy therapist. The therapist stated that the right and left hemispheres of my brain were disconnected from one another, that my mind was not connected to my brain, and that my throat chakra was spinning in the wrong direction. This was causing my fifth chakra to deflect any energy that was attempting to come to my pituitary, pineal, and adrenal glands; thus resulting in poor metabolism, hormone imbalance, and symptoms of depression, which also caused my thyroid to not function properly.

The therapist intuitively detected hidden fears coming from past events that were registering as trauma in the second and third chakras. I learned basic communication do's-and-don'ts when I felt like I was in conflict. I became non-reactive, yet present for solving the problem. I began to learn how to change the energy of the situation non-verbally by using meditation and visualization, and I noticed how it magically eased the situation on the human level and made communication clearer and easier for me to make other veterans to get comfortable enough to want to listen and take part in the group sessions.

I have approached the subject of "applying metaphysics in Holistic Life Coaching" by investigating the metaphysical teachings of Dr. Masters in general, and other methods of treatment specifically, from a variety of different sources. There is no question that sexual abuse and sexual trauma leave deep wounds that affect not only sexuality, but can compromise our basic identity and sense of self. And of the many faces of trauma, perhaps none is more debilitating than the feelings of shame and dirtiness. These feelings can cause us to "withdraw," to hide, or to act out in ways such as having experiences of promiscuity making us feel worse or even putting us in harm's way.

The basic tool we have in healing trauma of whatever kind is to find a way to "feel through" these internal states. When we free the vast potential of energy that is locked in trauma, we can assimilate these energies and feelings into our being and wholeness. My decision to go forward was based on the importance of addressing sexual trauma because it affects so many of us.

By even conservative estimates, worldwide, one in four persons has been sexually assaulted in childhood. In the USA, there are some 65 million in that category, potentially 1.5 billion in the world. If you are a woman, the chances are even greater. When you go into a supermarket to shop, look around you and realize that as many as one in four people there have been sexually assaulted as children. Whether you live in a small town or a large city, as you walk down any street on any ordinary day, you can be sure you are not alone. Know that you are not alone!

All of these estimates, however large, are only part of the story. First of all, they are numbers and tell nothing about the human suffering. In addition, many people are raped as adults and it is possible to be sexually traumatized by events that are not "supposed" to be traumatic! For example, it is possible that gynecological procedures -- when performed roughly and insensitively -- can cause the vital organs and energy systems in our pelvis and abdominal organs to go into a kind of "shock" not unlike what happens in sexual assault. This includes even roughly-administered thermometers and enemas in childhood.

Though not politically correct, abortions can be, and frequently are, traumatizing, as are other invasive surgeries performed in sexual and internal organs. In some ways, we need to be concerned about the cause of our loss of vitality and capacity for erotic connection and pleasure. But the remedy to heal and to restore access to these precious creative energies is what needs to be foremost, not the cause!

Speaking from experience, metaphysics helped me come a long way. That is why I firmly believe that my becoming a Holistic Life Coach will affect society in a much needed way as I continue to interact with veterans on a daily basis.

BIBLIOGRAPHY

AllAboutLifeChallenges.org. (2002 - 2012). *All About Life Challenges*. Retrieved from AllAboutGOD.com .

Baker-Eddy, M. (1934). *Science and Health with Key to the Scriptures*. Christian Science Board of Directors.

Brennan, T. (August 2003). *The Transmission of Affect*. Ithaca, New York: Cornell University Press.

Burns, D. (1989). *The Feeling Good Handbook*. Norfolk, VA: Plume.

Co, A. H. (1913. Print.). *Holy Bible. King James Version*. Philadelphia: A.J. Holman Co.

Cohen, R. (1987). *Rape Trauma Syndrome*. Retrieved from http://psychologytoday.psychtests.com/articles/mentalhealth/rapedev.html

Dale, C. (2009). *The Subtle Body: An Encyclopedia of Your Energetic Anatomy.* Sounds True, Incorporated.

Detweiler, N. (2005). *Welcome to the Pathway to Ascensiion.* Richmond, VA: Copyright © 2001-2009 Nancy B. Detweiler. Retrieved from Pathway to Ascension:
http://www.pathwaytoascension.com/bible5.html

Detweiler, N. B. (1997). *A New Age Christian: My Spiritual Journey.* Richmond, VA: Bridging the Gap Ministries

Driessen, A. (2003). *Connecting with YOur Multidimensional Self and Your Longing for Happiness.* Ebook.

Ellis, E. M. (1983). *Queendom.* Retrieved from http://www.queendom.com/articles/articles.htm?a=5&p=post_traumatic_stress_disorder:
http://www.queendom.com/articles/articles.htm?a=5&p=rape_trauma_syndrome

Foundation, T. N. (1995-2012). *TeensHealth.* Retrieved from

http://teenshealth.org/teen/kh_misc/about.html:
http://teenshealth.org/teen/safety/safebasics/rape_w
hat_to_do.html

Grant, R. (1998-1999). *Trauma May Open Door to
Spirituality.* Retrieved from PTSD Support
Services: http://www.ptsdsupport.net/gazette.html

Levine PhD, P. (1976). *"Waking the Tiger -
Healing Trauma,."* Berkeley, CA: North Atlantic
Books.

Levine PhD, P. (2008). *The Handling of Sexual
Trauma.* Retrieved from Extatica:
http://www.extatica.com/articles/Levine_P_Healin
gSacredWound_1.htm

Masters PhD, P. L. (1989). *Masters Degree Level
Lesson, Vol#1 Pg 18.* Board of Directors of the
International Metaphysical Ministry. Retrieved
from International Metaphysical Ministry:
http://www.immsite.com/imm-basic-metaphysical-
tenets.html

Masters PhD, P. L. (2010). *International
Metaphysical Ministry.* Retrieved from University

of Metaphysics: http://www.immsite.com/imm-basic-metaphysical-tenets.html

Renner. (1988). *Mental Health Articles: Rape Trauma Syndrome.* Retrieved from http://psychologytoday.psychtests.com/articles/mentalhealth/rapedev.html

Reque-Dragicevic, B. (2008). *Close to Home, A Soldiers Guide to Returning From War.* iUniverse. Retrieved from Healing Combat Trauma.

Rhoades, G. F. (2005, November 1). *Trauma and Dissociation in a Cross-Cultural Perspective, Not Just a North American Phenomenom* (Vols. Volume 4, Numbers 1/2 and 3/4,). (G. F. Rhoades, Ed.) Haworth Press, inc. Retrieved from http://www.actualfreedom.com.au/sundry/map.htm and http://www.actualfreedom.com.au/library/topics/dissociation.htm

Tansley, D. (1977). *Dimensions of Radionics* . Beekman Books Inc .

Woolger, R. J. (1996). *Past Life Therapy, Trauma Release and the Body.* Retrieved from rogerwoolger.com: http://www.rogerwoolger.com/pastlife.html

Woolger, R. J. (2010). *Healing Your Past Lives: Exploring the Many Lives of the Soul.* Sounds True, Incorporated; Pap/Com edition.

APPENDIX

For almost thirty years, I carried my deep dark secret. It caused me to lose myself, my self-esteem, my hopes, my dreams, relationships, friends, and family, etc. The worst part was I could never have another child.

People don't realize that sexual trauma is not a diagnosis or a mental health condition in and of itself, or that it is not surprising that we have a wide range of emotional responses. I began to notice the differences in my behavior -- feeling depressed; having intense, sudden emotional responses to things; feeling angry or irritable all the time; trouble falling or staying asleep; bad dreams or nightmares; trouble staying focused, often finding my mind wandering; having a hard time remembering things; drinking to excess or using drugs daily, getting drunk or "high" to cope with memories or unpleasant feelings, drinking to fall asleep; feeling on edge or "jumpy" all the time; not feeling safe; going out of your way to avoid reminders of the trauma; trouble trusting others, feeling alone or not connected to others; abusive relationships; trouble with employers or authority figures; sexual issues; chronic pain; weight and eating problems; and having stomach or bowel problems (which I still suffer with).

For me, I would compare it to wondering in the desert with no escape, or millions of cars driving around in my head. One would never be able to imagine what it would feel like unless you have experienced it, to have to leave your employment that you love, and all of your hopes and dreams of becoming a surgeon being lost forever. I didn't acknowledge the effects that military sexual trauma was having on my life.

After years of not recognizing the emotional effects of my experience, I told a VA practitioner about it and changed my life for the better. I had already tried drugs and alcohol; group counseling; PTSD awareness training; Veteran Administration's individual counseling for many years; candle magic, crystal and gemstone magic; numerology; herbology and herbal remedies; Native American healing beliefs; prescribed pharmaceuticals; Western medicine; chiropractic care; New Age healing techniques such as chakra cleansing many times; nutritional education; self-help books; and almost any other suggestion by any health care worker.

I still couldn't fall asleep. I couldn't remain asleep without waking up repeatedly during the night. And I was plagued by repeated traumatic nightmares every night. Sleep was my enemy and I fought it every night, waking up exhausted and tired.

I obsessed about sleep because I was always in sleep deficit. I would get very distressed if I stayed up late, yet couldn't seem to go to bed until late because I dreaded the nightmares. I wouldn't take naps during the day because it would make getting to sleep more difficult at night. The things that I tried helped very little.

I was open to alternative healing and had tried many things, but nothing had truly brought me the relief I wanted and needed. I was willing to give anything a try. In addition to my resentment against men, I just felt lost and alone.

Even though I feel completely overwhelmed right now, I deeply and completely accept that. Even though I don't want to think about what happened, I choose to allow myself to heal anyway. Even though I am nervous that this meditation won't work, I choose to be surprisingly calm and confident.

I managed not to wake up last night and slept the whole night through, but that was just that night. I had to keep giving myself affirmations, and telling myself that it was possible for me to recover. Every day, I noticed that I wanted to pick up my old emotional trauma/baggage.

I kept revisiting my trauma over and over. I wanted to find the old baggage because it has been with me for so long, it's comfortable, it's what I know, and I felt awkward and exposed without it. I recognized what I was doing and did some self-talk and self-encouragement, and was able to just let myself be without trying to re-find any of my emotional baggage by treating myself with love and compassion. Even though I have been though more than most people will ever understand, I'm learning to deeply and completely accept myself.

Even though I resent the fact that I had to go through all this, it's just not fair and I don't deserve it, I deeply and completely accept myself. Even though sleep is not safe for me, I am trying to allow myself to realize that all this happened a long time ago.

I Am understanding that repair of the physical and emotional damage that afflicts man in general can be achieved through growth and recognition of each of our own particular I Am Self, or God-Head.

Accepting this as my truth and a way to heal myself, I started to combine spirituality, metaphysics, prayer and meditation as a way to steer myself away from what I was going through, feeling and living with on a daily basis.